Myrrh Essential Oil

Benefits, Properties, Applications, Studies & Recipes

by Ann Sullivan

Published in USA by:

Ann Sullivan
217 N. Seacrest Blvd #9
Boynton Beach
FL 33425

© Copyright 2015

ISBN-13: 978-1545427477
ISBN-10: 154542747X

TABLE OF CONTENTS

Introduction

What are essential oils, and how might they be used for therapeutic purposes?

Essential oils are ultra-potent oils, extracted from plants and flowers that have been utilized in medicine for centuries. Presently, they're most commonly used to supplement pharmaceutical medication, but they can also be an effective alternative to pharmaceuticals in the event that you don't have access to them. Before you dismiss essential oils as a means to support the body's natural defenses against injuries and illness, take a look at the historical evidence of the oils' medicinal competence in practice. Your average age-old medical text will demonstrate that essential oils, herbs, and plenty of other natural ingredients have, for thousands of years, successfully enhanced immune function to meet and defeat any number of ailments and injuries. Though traditional medicine is considered "alternative" now, it was once the gold standard. And, frankly, perhaps it still should be, as these natural age-tested remedies can fortify the body's battlements against everything from simple maladies, like headaches, cuts and bruises, to serious diseases, like cancer.

Essential oils are deemed "essential," because the oils are composed of the "essence" of the plant. The difference between essential oils and other oils – like olive oil or vegetable oil, for instance – is that essential oils have high volatility and reduced fixation, which results in faster evaporation, enabling their popular use in aromatherapy. Even at high temperatures, olive and vegetable oils don't evaporate.

Essential oils are especially necessary when it comes to a major natural or man-made disaster or some potential viral outbreak. In these types of dire situations, you may not have quick access (or any access at all) to your standard pharmaceutical supply; so essential oils, along with other alternative medicines, will be your go-to health aids in the case of social collapse, viral outbreak or devastating natural disaster. When medical access is null and void, alternatives to our modern-day standard are the only chance we have to keep pathogens at bay.

You probably don't realize that you already use essential oils every day. They're in perfumes, shampoos, soaps, ointments...they're even used in furniture polish. Why are they found in so many aromatic products? Well, basically, because essential oils are super concentrated aromatic liquids, so their scent is remarkably strong. Let's put this into perspective: to steam tea, you use a few leaves of peppermint or juniper; to produce a single ounce of essential oil, five whole pounds of peppermint or juniper leaves are required. Some sources claim that to produce twelve pounds of essential oil would necessitate an acre of peppermint, juniper, or any other oil you're looking to produce en masse. Unlike vegetable oil, you don't often find concentrated therapeutic-grade essential oils sold by the tubload; instead the oils are often sold in easily carried small, dark bottles, perfect for your everyday carry bag.

Why myrrh, you ask? Well, in order to get you quickly up to speed on this most essential of oils, below we've provided a condensed synopsis of myrrh, after which we'll outline in greater detail the oil's history, properties, and common therapeutic uses, so that you – the consumer – might have a better understanding of the oil's benefits and applications. We've even provided supportive remedies for pure myrrh, as well as blended recipes that incorporate the valuable oil. Chapter 3 will further detail past scientific research on myrrh essential oil.

Now, let's get down to it.

Essential Oil 101: the Basics of Myrrh

Summary: Myrrh, or Commiphora myrrha, has been used for thousands of years by the Ancient Egyptians and by the Arabians, primarily to support skin conditions. The antioxidant properties of myrrh effectively benefit everything from wrinkles to chapped or cracked skin. Myrrh is also full of sesquiterpenes, which aid the pituitary, hypothalamus and amygdala, all of which deeply affects emotions. This results in an uplifting and restorative sense of being. With such estimable properties, it's no wonder that myrrh was gifted to the baby Jesus, alongside gold and frankincense.

Description: Myrrh oil is commonly extracted through steam distillation. The resin is most often used. The oil is golden in color, medium in consistency, and has a somewhat strong warm and woody scent.

Uses: Beyond those applications previously mentioned, additional uses for myrrh essential oil include supporting the body's defenses against athlete's foot, chapped skin, halitosis, itching, ringworm, amenorrhea, bronchitis, dysmenorrhea, gums, oral hygiene, toothache, colds, flu, cough, cuts, wounds, diarrhea, hemorrhoids, dermatitis, indigestion, stomachache, yeast infection and other skin issues. When it comes to mood and emotion, myrrh essential oil can help relieve stress by providing an uplifting sense of being.

Properties: Antioxidant, anti-inflammatory, antiseptic, antibacterial, antifungal, antispasmodic, anticarcinogenic, astringent, decongestant, sedative, stimulant, analgesic, vulnerary, stomachic, carminative, expectorant, vasodilator, tonic, and stimulant properties.

Application: Use neat or undiluted. You can apply topically, inhale directly, diffuse or use as a dietary supplement.

Safety Precautions: Myrrh has been approved by the FDA for internal consumption and so can be used as a dietary supplement. However, if pregnant, breastfeeding or diabetic, consult a physician before using this oil.

Fun facts: Myrrh is derived from the Arabic word for "bitter," which is "murr."

Mentioned over 150 times in the Bible, myrrh has been

valued for thousands of years, even making an appearance in the ancient Egyptian medical text, Ebers Papyrus, which includes 700 therapeutic remedies from 1550 BC.

One of the many traditional applications for this oil was to uplift. Pregnant women were often anointed with the oil to improve their mood.

Chapter 1:
Benefits of Myrrh Essential Oil

Myrrh essential oil offers a number of therapeutic benefits; but you may be wondering what these benefits are. In this chapter, we'll take a closer look at the history of myrrh and its many uses.

Cultivation of Myrrh

Myrrh is a scented resin and natural gum that is derived from the thorny tree of the genera Commiphora. Although there are plenty of species branching from this genera, Commiphora myrrha is the most common source of essential oil and originates in eastern Ethiopia, Yemen, Eritrea, and Somalia. Like frankincense, myrrh resin or gum bleeds through tree wounds, when there is a break through the bark and into the sapwood. To harvest myrrh, the poor trees must be stabbed and bled repeatedly in order to extract the resin, which, to begin with, quickly coagulates and is waxy and yellow opaque or clear but, following the extraction, becomes glossy, tough, and darker in color as time passes. White streaks, as well, often appear in the resin. Though Commiphora myrrha/Commiphora molmol (synonymous) is harvested most commonly today, the famed Commiphora gileadensis is most likely to have produced the biblically referenced myrrh, also called the Balm of Gilead and Balsam of Mecca, which originates in the Arabian Peninsula and Eastern Mediterranean.

A History of Myrrh

Myrrh is derived from the Hebrew "mor" and the Arabic "mur," both of which mean "bitter." In ancient times, camel caravans traveled overland to trade myrrh that was produced by the Nabataeans in southern Arabia. It was taken from there to the capital city, Petra, where after it was transported to areas throughout the Mediterranean.

The resin has a long history of use in everything from medicine to perfumery, and incense to winery. As a medicine, the oleo gum resin was used to dress wounds, while the fragrant use of myrrh is recorded innumerable times in the Old Testament, where it is oft quoted as being used in perfumery which was said to have been intoxicating. One recording from Genesis 37:25, for example, states where the resin originated, "As they sat down to eat their meal, they looked up and saw a caravan of Ishmaelites coming from Gilead. Their camels were loaded with spices, balm and myrrh, and they were on their way to take them down to Egypt," while Exodus 30:23 suggests the value of myrrh at the time of Moses, "Take the following fine spices: 500 shekels of liquid myrrh, half as much (that is, 250 shekels) of fragrant cinnamon… You shall make of these a holy anointing oil." And, of course, myrrh's most famed reference in the Bible is that of its gifting to the Christ Child from the Three Wise Men. Perhaps, not so well remembered, is that myrrh came full circle in the life of Christ; Jesus was offered myrrh a second and final time, right before his crucifixion, assumedly to help sedate the pain: "Then they offered him wine mixed with myrrh, but he did not take it" (Mark 15:23). This was a traditional gesture by the Romans – the offering of drugged wine – to help ease the suffering of crucifixion. According to scripture, Christ refused the gesture, in order to feel the full extent of his suffering.

Christian literature is not the only ancient record of myrrh's early prominence. The ancient Greeks had long considered myrrh to be a potent aphrodisiac. This application of myrrh is illustrated in the Greek myth of Myrrha. Myrrha was a young woman, in love with the king of Cyprus, who just so happened to be her father. Despite the fact that she harbored a forbidden love, she accepted no suitors and, instead, chose to commit suicide. Before she was able, her intentions were discovered by her nurse, who persuaded Myrrha to forego her own death in order to seduce her father. The nurse suggested she could help her in the attempt and did so, assisting Myrrha in hiding her identity and succeeding in the affair, by keeping to the shadows. However, the king was curious about his lover's identity, and one day, he lit a lamp, only to discover the awful truth. As the king drew his sword to murder his own daughter, she fled and wandered the Ethiopian deserts for nine months, where she began to have contractions, for she was pregnant with her father's son (and her brother). At her wit's end, Myrrha begged the gods for mercy, and the mercy they provided was turning Myrrha into a tree. Helped along by the goddess of childbirth, the tree gave birth to Adonis.

This myth claims that the resin of the tree is actually Myrrha's tears, the only human fragment left of her mortality. These tears serve as an aphrodisiac and, in fact, myrrh resin has long been used in Sumerian perfumes and incense for just that reason.

Additional links to foreign gods include the ancient Egyptian lunar goddess of fertility, Isis, who is a significant female archetype, representing energy and receptiveness (frankincense, meanwhile, was considered masculine, representing active energy). Myrrh incense was often burned at high noon in Egypt to celebrate Isis.

Ancient China, as well, found innumerable uses for myrrh. Chinese medicine believed its properties moved the blood (modern research supports this use), which, in turn, fortified the heart, liver, spleen, and uterus. Similarly to frankincense, the Chinese thereby applied it to support such health issues as uterine conditions, menopause, and menstrual issues, like dysmenorrhea and amenorrhea, as well as circulatory and inflammatory problems, including arthritis and rheumatism. Ayuverdic medicine touted myrrh's rejuvenatory and tonic properties, and used it similarly to the Chinese for circulatory issues and rheumatism, as well as for nervous system disorders.

Myrrh is used in modern western medicine primarily as an antiseptic in relation to oral health and hygiene. As an ingredient in toothpastes, gargles, and mouthwashes, myrrh strengthens gums and protects against gum disease, while its analgesic properties help relieve toothaches. Myrrh is also an ingredient in certain skin healing salves to help accelerate the healing process of minor abrasions and is recommended as a liniment for aches, sprains, and bruises.

Myrrh was also used in a variety of religious rituals. Ancient Egyptians applied myrrh to the embalming of mummies, while the First and Second Temples of Jerusalem utilized myrrh as a consecrated incense. The holy anointing oil was also blended to bless kings, high priests, and the Tabernacle. In Islamic tradition, myrrh was used as a house fumigant. It is mentioned in the Encyclopedia of Islamic Herbal Medicine that "the Messenger of Allah stated, 'Fumigate your houses with al-shih, murr, and sa'tar.'"

According to the book of Esther, the oil was also used to "purify" women. They were anointed with the oil for six months – and other "sweet odors" for six months more – in order to be presented to King Ahasuerus, the king of

Persia.

With so many ancient uses for myrrh, it's no wonder that it remains, to this day, a sacred and ritualistic aromatic resin and essential oil.

Chemical Components

In order to generate the essential oil from myrrh, the resin must be steam distilled. This results in the oil's key chemical components, which are primarily limonene, alpha pinene, eugenol, acetic acid, formic acid, cadinene, cuminaldehyde, heerabolene, cresol, and sesquiterpenes.

Main Properties of Myrrh Essential Oil

Along with the properties previously mentioned in the introduction, myrrh oil possesses antioxidant, anti-inflammatory, antiseptic, antibacterial, antifungal, antispasmodic, anticarcinogenic, astringent, decongestant, sedative, stimulant, analgesic, vulnerary, stomachic, carminative, expectorant, vasodilator, tonic, and stimulant properties. With such a versatile range, myrrh is well equipped to fight off any pathogen in the body's path.

Myrrh, as mentioned, is composed of limonene, alpha pinene, eugenol, acetic acid, formic acid, cadinene, cuminaldehyde, heerabolene, cresol, and sesquiterpenes. These components are what instill the enormously beneficial properties within myrrh essential oil. We'll outline these properties below.

Antioxidant

Anything high in antioxidants – whether fruit, beans, or essential oils – is a powerful advocate for your body. Antioxidants both protect against free radicals and repair their damage. What are free radicals? Free radicals are destructive chemicals that invade your body, produced by substances both inside and out. Some free radicals (or oxidants) form through normal bodily reactions, like inflammation, metabolism and aerobic respiration. Other free radicals form outside the body, but enter it due to exposure. These include harmful pollutants, toxins, smoking, alcohol, X-rays, and UV rays, to name a few.

Although our bodies produce their own antioxidants, these often become damaged as we grow older; thus, introducing antioxidants into our bodies allows these nutrients and enzymes to assist in chemical reactions which destroy the oxidants or free radicals. Myrrh essential oil is a moderate antioxidant, aiming to detox the body of free radicals that lead to disease.

Anti-inflammatory

External or internal inflammation can be reduced through the use of myrrh essential oil. For instance, if you or your patient has swollen fingers from arthritis or a swollen knee from a sport's injury, oral application of myrrh essential oil may decrease irritation or redness, while also soothing the pain that accompanies inflammation.

Antiseptic

The antiseptic properties of myrrh essential oil can be reaped topically, applied directly to wounds, or even through burning; the smoke from the oil may help destroy airborne germs. Internal use will help keep the wounds from becoming infections, while external use will support the body's natural function in inhibiting tetanus.

Antibacterial

Myrrh's antibacterial properties make it a powerful protectant against diseases produced by bacteria, such as oral, digestive and urinary tract bacterial infection. What's great is that, unlike some prescription drugs, myrrh has no ill effects on bodily health or on the healthy natural flora that exists within the stomach and intestines.

Antifungal

While bacteria and viruses are plenty evil, fungi commonly lead to the most deadly infections, whether external or internal. Your ears, throat and nose are the most likely to become infected by fungi, the infections of which can be both excruciating and unsightly. If left untreated, fungal infections can kill, as they may spread to the brain. Myrrh essential oil protects against these infections and more and is particularly effective against skin infections.

Antispasmodic

The antispasmodic properties of myrrh essential oil make it beneficial to such health issues as chronic coughing and other respiratory conditions, along with surgical processes, such as colonoscopy and gastroscopy.

Anticarcinogenic

Myrrh essential oil has been shown to act as an anticarcinogen. An anticarcinogen counters those carcinogens which can potentially develop into cancer. Whereas anticarcinomas are used to treat cancer cells after cancer has developed, anticarcinogenics are natural defenses against the development of cancer.

Astringent

For those who do not know what an astringent is, it's a chemical compound that shrinks body tissues, which means it can aid skin issues and irritations, everything from acne to insect bites. The astringent property of myrrh essential oil benefits everything from skin to hair to gums to muscles to intestines. As an astringent, myrrh is an anti-agent, combating muscle loss through the ability to strengthen. This astringent property also mean that myrrh can support wound and cut bleeding

Decongestant

As a decongestant, myrrh essential oil can alleviate nasal congestion in the upper respiratory tract.

Sedative

Myrrh sedates and calms by reducing anxiety, excitement or irritability. Though sedatives, alone, do not alleviate pain, they do calm the patient, making them less stressed and more compliant.

Stimulant

Stimulants are often referred to as "uppers." This is because they produce mental or physical improvements or temporary enhancements of your bodily functions. For instance, you may grow more alert and awake or quicker on your feet after using a stimulant. Myrrh essential oil can provide this temporary boost in mental and physical function, especially when it comes to the immune system.

Analgesic

As an analgesic, myrrh essential oil supports pain relief, acting on the central nervous system to fortify the body's natural defenses against inflammation and supporting relief from pain receptor sensation.

Vulnerary

Whether you wish to address an ulcer, a cut, or any internal or external wound, myrrh essential oil can be diluted with a skin cream and applied to expedite the process of healing while also protecting the wound from becoming infected.

Stomachic

As a stomachic, myrrh improves stomach function, boosts appetite, and helps to tone the stomach. The oil helps control the stomach's bile, acid and gastric liquids.

Carminative

By supporting the reduction of excess gas buildup and/or removal of gas from the intestines, myrrh essential oil provides relief from abdominal pain, excess sweating, and uncomfortable indigestion.

Expectorant

Throat or respiratory infections can be relieved through the use of myrrh essential oil. Acting as an expectorant, myrrh breaks up and helps destroy the phlegm and mucus buildup that accompanies sinuses or respiratory infections. Inflamed throat and lungs – and, thus, coughing – can also be alleviated through the application of this oil.

Vasodilator

A vasodilator widens blood vessels by relaxing smooth muscle cells within the vessel walls. By dilating blood vessels, blood flow is increased, thereby decreasing blood pressure. Myrrh essential oil serves as a vasodilator and can therefore support the regulation of blood pressure.

Tonic

Myrrh essential oil benefits each of the body's systems, whether nervous, digestive, respiratory or excretory, making it an unbeatable general tonic. The oil also supports the immune system by helping the body absorb nutrients.

Stimulant

Stimulants are often referred to as "uppers." This is because they produce mental or physical improvements or temporary enhancements of your bodily functions. For instance, you may grow more alert and awake or quicker on your feet after using a stimulant. Myrrh essential oil can provide this temporary boost in mental and physical function, especially when it comes to the immune system.

Common Medicinal Uses

Traditionally used to enhance the body's defenses against skin issues, myrrh essential oil remains a significant derma support, protecting against a number of everyday problems, like chapped, dry, cracked, or sensitive skin, or more problematic conditions like eczema, acne, or dermatitis. Moreover, myrrh essential oil supports overall health, while relieving inflammation and pain. Let's take a closer look at the common uses for this oil.

Skin Health

Myrrh aids in skin health, particularly when it comes to inflammation. The chemical components of myrrh also help relieve wrinkles, infections, ulcers, and other skin imperfections, as they serve skin as an anti-inflammatory and an astringent. Additionally, the oil possesses antibacterial, antiseptic and antifungal properties that strengthen all skin types – oily or dry – by maintaining health of the derma. As a topical antiseptic, myrrh enhances your body's defenses against infections in wounds, burns and blisters.

Immune System Booster

Myrrh is a superb immune system support which boosts circulation and increases white blood cell count. The oil is akin to an immune shield braced to fight off inflammatory, fungal, and bacterial strains that attack the immune system. With such strong armor, this immune stimulant will ensure that your body is better prepared to protect against deadly infections.

Women's Health

Myrrh can significantly benefit women who experience painful cramps, as it helps relieve muscle contraction during menstruation. If you commonly experience painful or irregular periods that impact your daily life, a myrrh application can both help sedate the pain and uplift the spirit.

Infections

Myrrh essential oil is also a good combatant against infectious diseases, such as fungal meningitis and urinary tract infections. Moreover, myrrh has the ability to control fevers which sometimes accompany these infections.

Cardiovascular Health

Cardiovascular health can be maintained through the use of myrrh essential oil, in that it helps to reduce bad cholesterol (LDL) and boost good cholesterol (HDL), resulting in better cardiovascular health. The oil is also a vasodilator, which means it increases blood flow, thereby decreasing blood pressure. The oil's antioxidant properties and its ability to facilitate the dissolution of cholesterol that accumulates in arteries enable its support of cardiovascular issues, like heart disease or atherosclerosis.

Blood Circulation

An application of myrrh essential oil produces stimulant responses in the body, among them, increased blood circulation. When the oil vapor touches the olfactory nerve ends, the pulse quickens and blood circulates, providing more oxygen to the body's organs, including the brain, which promotes cognitive function. The oxygenation to the brain and other organs also serves to protect against degenerative diseases, like Alzheimer's.

Oral Health & Hair Health

If you have unhealthy hair, myrrh is just what you need to give your hair's gloss and strength a boost. As opposed to the harsh, dry, damaging chemicals in dandruff shampoos, myrrh is an all-natural alternative that serves your skin and hair by providing it with the proteins and vitamins essential to hair growth. Myrrh also strengthens gums, promoting oral health and hygiene.

Safety Precautions & Common Applications

Safety

Certain adverse effects may evolve when using pure essential oils. Some essential oils should not be used when pregnant, for example, as they may cause miscarriage. Allergic reactions, too, may occur, especially when applied topically. Always administer an allergy test before committing fully to topical application. When used with other medications, essential oils may react negatively. If you are on any current prescription medications or have a chronic illness, such as high blood pressure, epilepsy or liver disease, then researching the effects of essential oils against your own personal medical history will eliminate any potentially problematic issues.

Myrrh has been approved by the FDA for internal consumption and so can be used as a dietary supplement. If you are pregnant, use with caution and at the discretion of your physician. If you have sensitive skin, dilute heavily and test before extensive use. Otherwise, use neat (undiluted) or dilute 1:1 with a carrier oil. You can apply topically, diffuse or use as a dietary supplement.

Blends

Oftentimes, essential oils are manufactured as blends of several pure oils. For instance, the Protective Blend of certain brands is a mix of cinnamon, clove, rosemary, and eucalyptus. This blend can be used to boost the immune system to help support colds, viruses and flus. The downside to blends is that the more oils added to the mix, the higher the probability your patient may react negatively to the blend if he/she is prone to allergies. There is also the possibility of phototoxicity when working with blends, particularly if they include citrus oils. Be sure to read your labels before administering.

Regardless of these possible effects, essential oils are a viable option for supporting a number of conditions. Those looking to support or maintain their own personal health, or that of their families', should become educated on the uses of essential oils, their natural remedies and the methods of application. Only then can you begin building your kit of essential oils for survival.

Chapter 2:
Recipes for Myrrh Essential Oil

In this chapter, we'll offer various recipes for myrrh essential oil, both for pure myrrh applications and blends. For pure applications, we've provided the appropriate dosage and method of administration to support specific ailments, from cancer to wrinkles. When it comes to blends, herbalists and aromatherapists often combine myrrh essential oil with thyme, frankincense, tea tree, lavender, patchouli, and sandalwood essential oils. We'll offer some fantastic blending options in the second half of this chapter.

Pure Applications

Abandonment

Whenever you're feeling abandoned, pour a drop of myrrh essential oil into your hands, rub your palms together, cup them over your nose, and breathe deeply in and out for several minutes. For added support, diffuse throughout the home.

Brain Stimulant

To help stimulate the brain, apply topically, using myrrh essential oil neat or diluted in a 1:1 ratio with a carrier oil and massaging into the temples, forehead, back of the neck, and the reflex points of the feet. You can also add a drop or two to your drinking water and take internally.

Cancer

Help strengthen the body's natural defenses against cancer by using myrrh essential oil neat or diluting in a 1:1 ratio with a carrier oil; then apply topically, massaging into the reflex points of the feet or over the affected area. You can also diffuse throughout the home for overall health.

Congestion

Clear congestion by using myrrh essential oil neat or diluting in a 1:1 ratio with a carrier oil, then apply topically, massaging it over the affected area. You can also inhale the oil directly for nasal congestion, diffuse throughout the home, or gargle with warm salt water.

Dysentery

Support the body's natural defenses against dysentery by using myrrh essential oil neat or diluting in a 1:1 ratio with a carrier oil and massaging it in a counter-clockwise direction into the lower abdomen and lower back, over the area of the intestines, and into the reflex points of the feet. This will fight infection, inflammation and diarrhea.

Fear

To help eliminate unwarranted fear, use myrrh essential oil neat or dilute in a 1:1 ratio with a carrier oil and apply topically, massaging over the solar plexus and the heart. You can also administer aromatically, diffusing throughout the home or inhaling directly from the bottle.

Gum Disease

To combat gum disease, add a drop or two of myrrh essential oil to your daily brushing regimen. Brush as normal.

Hashimoto's Thyroiditis

To support healthy thyroid function, pour a drop of myrrh essential oil into your hands, rub your palms together, cup them over your nose, and breathe deeply in and out for several minutes. For added support, diffuse throughout the home.

Hepatitis

Strengthen the body's natural defenses against hepatitis by diffusing or steaming two drops of myrrh essential oil in a pan of water. Then remove the steaming pan from the stove, pour into a bowl, place a towel over your head and inhale. If you don't feel it's done its job the first time, you can reheat that same water and use it once more without adding additional oil. You can also use myrrh essential oil neat or dilute in a 1:1 ratio with a carrier oil and apply topically, massaging over the body and into the soles of the feet every day.

Hypothyroidism

Support healthy thyroid function by diffusing myrrh essential oil. You can also apply topically by using myrrh essential oil neat or diluting in a 1:1 ratio with a carrier oil and massaging over the thyroid.

Infection

To fight off infection, use myrrh essential oil neat or dilute in a 1:1 ratio with a carrier oil and apply topically to the affected area or to the soles of the feet. You can also diffuse throughout the room or take internally, whichever application is more appropriate to your specific infection.

Inflammation

Calm inflammation by using myrrh essential oil neat or diluting in a 1:1 ratio with a carrier oil, then apply topically, massaging the oil over the affected area towards the heart. For added support, add a drop to your drinking water and take internally or diffuse throughout the home.

Liver Support

Support liver function by using myrrh essential oil neat or diluting in a 1:1 ratio with a carrier oil; then apply topically, massaging over the affected area and into the reflex points of the feet. You can also place a drop in your drinking water and take internally on a daily basis.

Pain

General pain can be eased by using myrrh essential oil neat or diluting in a 1:1 ratio with a carrier oil; apply topically, massaging over the affected area and the reflex points of the feet.

Parasites

To combat parasites, take orally in either capsules or add a drop to your drinking water. You can also apply externally, using myrrh essential oil neat or diluting in a 1:1 ratio with a carrier oil and massaging into the soles of the feet or over the affected area.

Prostate Support

To support the prostate, use myrrh essential oil neat or dilute in a 1:1 ratio with a carrier oil and apply topically over the affected area and into the reflex points of the feet on a regular basis. You can also take internally, by adding a drop to your drinking water regularly throughout the day or adding 5-6 drops in a veggie capsule and consuming after each meal.

Skin (Chapped, Dry, Cracked, Sensitive, Eczema, Acne, Dermatitis, etc.)

Myrrh essential oil can support all types of skin conditions. Use myrrh essential oil neat or dilute in a 1:1 ratio with a carrier oil and apply topically to the affected area. You can also add a drop of myrrh to your daily skin regimen.

Stretch Marks

Protect against and reduce the appearance of stretch marks by massaging myrrh essential oil neat or diluted in a 1:1 ratio with a carrier oil and apply directly over the affected area, two or three times daily.

Sunscreen

For an effective sunscreen, add 4-5 drops of myrrh essential oil to regular skin lotion. Apply every two hours when you're exposed to the sun.

Thyroid Healthy

Support healthy thyroid function by diffusing myrrh essential oil throughout the home. You can also apply topically by using myrrh essential oil neat or diluting in a 1:1 ratio with a carrier oil and massaging over the thyroid.

Trust

Promote trust by diffusing myrrh essential oil throughout the home. You can also apply topically, using myrrh essential oil neat or diluting in a 1:1 ratio with a carrier oil; then massage into the solar plexus, over the heart, or in a full-body massage. Additionally, you can pour a drop of myrrh essential oil into your hands, rub your palms together, cup them over your nose, and breathe deeply in and out for several minutes.

Tumors

To protect against tumors or reduce their growth, use myrrh essential oil neat or dilute in a 1:1 ratio with a carrier oil and apply topically to the affected area or into the reflex points of the feet.

Ulcer (Duodenal)

Target ulcers internally by placing a drop of myrrh essential oil in each glass of drinking water or add 2-3 drops to a veggie capsule and take after each meal.

Ulcer (Skin)

Target skin ulcers externally by using myrrh essential oil neat or diluting in a 1:1 ratio with a carrier oil and applying topically, massaging into the affected area, and the reflex points of the feet.

Vaginal Infection

Strengthen the body's natural defenses against vaginal infection by external application. Use myrrh essential oil neat or dilute in a 1:1 ratio with a carrier oil and apply topically to the lower abdomen, massaging over the groin, but avoiding the genitals up to three times daily. Take care to use caution.

Weeping Wounds

Help accelerate the healing process of weeping wounds by using myrrh essential oil neat or diluting in a 1:1 ratio with a carrier oil. Then apply topically to affected area up to three times, daily.

Wrinkles

Protect against wrinkles or reduce their appearance by using myrrh essential oil neat or diluting in a 1:1 ratio with a carrier oil and massaging over the affected area. You can also add a drop or two to your daily skincare regimen. Be careful around the eyes.

Blend

Anti-Aging Salve

Ingredients

- 5 drops Geranium Essential Oil
- 5 drops Frankincense Essential Oil
- 5 drops Myrrh Essential Oil
- 5 drops Rosemary Essential Oil
- 5 drops Lemon Essential Oil
- 10 drops Rosehip Essential Oil
- 10 drops Carrot Seed Essential Oil
- 10 drops Sandalwood Essential Oil
- ½ cup Apricot Kernel Oil

Directions

To reduce the signs of skin aging, combine all ingredients in a small glass jar or container, blending well. After your evening facial routine, apply to areas of concern. Use as needed, blending well before each use.

Athlete's Foot

Ingredients

- 6 drops Myrrh Essential Oil

- 6 drops Thyme Essential Oil

- 8 drops Eucalyptus Essential Oil

- 10 drops Tea Tree Essential Oil

- 2 ounces Carrier Oil

Directions

In a small glass jar or container, mix all ingredients until well combined. To help relieve athlete's foot, apply 2-3 drops topically, twice a day or as needed. Continue consistent use for several weeks after the infection clears up, as fungal infections are stubborn and take a while to be eliminated completely.

Corns & Calluses

Ingredients

- 6 drops Myrrh Essential Oil

- 12 drops Lavender Essential Oil

- 2 ounces Sweet Almond Oil

Directions

In a small bowl or container, mix all ingredients until well combined. To relieve corns or calluses, apply topically, massaging into the affected area every day.

Hepatitis

Ingredients

- 4 drops Basil Essential Oil

- 4 drops Myrrh Essential Oil

- 4 drops Cypress Essential Oil

- 8 drops Coconut Oil

Directions

To support the body's natural defenses against hepatitis, place all ingredients into a small bowl or container and blend thoroughly then administer topically, massaging into the liver and into the reflex points of the hands and feet.

You can also place 2 drops of each essential oil into a "00" capsule, and ingest 1 capsule twice daily.

Hypothyroid Blend

Ingredients

- 12 drops Peppermint Essential Oil

- 12 drops Clove Bud Essential Oil

- 12 drops Lemongrass Essential Oil

- 10 drops Myrrh Essential Oil

- 1 Tbsp Coconut Oil

Directions

For thyroid support, combine all ingredients in a small glass bowl or container, blending well. Then apply topically, massaging over the thyroid three times daily.

Labor Inducer

Ingredients

- 2 drops Clary Sage Essential Oil

- 7 drops Myrrh Essential Oil

Directions

To help induce or speed labor, apply a single drop of clary sage to the reflex points in each ankle, while diffusing myrrh. Only use this method on or after your due date.

Nail Health

Ingredients

- 1 drop Wintergreen Essential Oil

- 2 drops Lemon Essential Oil

- 2 drops Myrrh Essential Oil

- 2 drops Frankincense Essential Oil

- 4 drops Wheat Germ

Directions

In a small jar or container, mix all ingredients until well combined. Two or three times a day, place a single drop of the blend on each nail and rub into the nail and cuticle to promote strong nails.

Ovarian Cyst

Ingredients

- 2 drops Thyme Essential Oil

- 2 drops Rosemary Essential Oil

- 5 drops Clary Sage Essential Oil

- 5 drops Myrrh Essential Oil

- 9 drops Frankincense Essential Oil

Directions

In a small bowl or container, mix all ingredients until well combined. Apply 1-3 drops on the respective reflex points on the anklebones on either side of the feet. You can also apply with a warm compress over the area of concern.

Respiratory Health

Ingredients

- 8 drops Myrrh Essential Oil
- 8 drops Frankincense Essential Oil
- 6 drops Eucalyptus Essential Oil
- 3 drops Pine Essential Oil
- 3 drops Rosemary Essential Oil
- 2 drops Peppermint Essential Oil
- 30 mL Jojoba Oil

Directions

To promote respiratory health and clear breathing, combine all ingredients in a small glass jar or bowl, blending well. Apply topically to the chest and the reflex points of the feet, breathing the aroma in deeply.

You can also eliminate the carrier oil and diffuse throughout the home.

Scar Salve

Ingredients

- 4 drops Patchouli Essential Oil

- 5 drops Myrrh Essential Oil

- 6 drops Lavender Essential Oil

- 8 drops Lemongrass Essential Oil

- 10 drops Helichrysum Essential Oil

- 1 ounce Carrier Oil

Directions

To fade the appearance of scars or protect against scarring, combine all ingredients in a small glass bowl or container, blending well. Apply topically to affected area.

Scar Salve II

Ingredients

- 2 drops Sandalwood Essential Oil

- 4 drops Lavender Essential Oil

- 6 drops Helichrysum Essential Oil

- 6 drops Myrrh Essential Oil

- 1 Tbsp Grapeseed Oil

Directions

To fade the appearance of scars or protect against scarring, combine all ingredients in a small glass bowl or container, blending well. Apply topically to affected area.

Sinuses

Ingredients

- 3 drops Rosemary Essential Oil

- 3 drops Oregano Essential Oil

- 3 drops Protective Blend Essential Oil

- 2 drops Myrrh Essential Oil

- 2 drops Frankincense Essential Oil

Directions

To clear sinuses, place all ingredients into a "00" capsule, and ingest 1 capsule 1-3 times a day or as needed. Continue taking for 2 days after symptoms subside.

Sunscreen

Ingredients

- 7 drops Myrrh Essential Oil

- 7 drops Helichrysum Essential Oil

- 1 ounce Carrier Oil

Instructions

For an effective sunscreen, place all ingredients into a bottle and shake. Apply every two hours when you're exposed to the sun.

Chapter 3:
Myrrh Essential Oil Studies

Many studies have been done on essential oils to uncover and prove their therapeutic qualities. In the case of the great number of myrrh studies, many of the properties attributed to the essential oil (noted in this book and elsewhere) are quite often validated through the research from accredited universities and published by reputable scientific journals. In this chapter, we'll discuss a small portion of these studies. It's important to note that our knowledge of essential oils is constantly evolving. Keep up with any recent research, as it may turn up even further valuable uses for these miracle oils.

Study 1 – Anticancer Properties (Breast Cancer)

In this study published by the Oncology Letters, the anticancer effects of myrrh essential oil were examined, with the following results: "The present study aimed to investigate the composition and potential anticancer activities of essential oils obtained from two species, myrrh and frankincense...The results indicated that the MCF-7 and HS-1 cell lines showed increased sensitivity to the myrrh and frankincense essential oils compared with the remaining cell lines. In addition, the anticancer effects of myrrh were markedly increased compared with those of frankincense, however, no significant synergistic effects were identified. The flow cytometry results indicated that apoptosis may be a major contributor to the biological efficacy of MCF-7 cells."

MCF-7 is a breast cancer cell line. When the cell line is broached by frankincense or myrrh essential oils, the result is cell death. In multicellular organisms, apoptosis is the process of programmed cell death. In the case of cancer, an insufficient amount of apoptosis results in an unmanageable growth of cancer cells, so the cell death stimulated by myrrh essential oil is necessary to control the cancer. The results of the study demonstrate that myrrh exhibited anticancer effects against the breast cancer cell line, indicating its efficacy in strengthening the body's defenses against breast cancer.

Reference:
http://www.ncbi.nlm.nih.gov/pubmed/24137478

http://www.ncbi.nlm.nih.gov/pmc/articles/PMC3796379/
pdf/ol-06-04-1140.pdf]

Study 2 – Anti-inflammatory Properties

In this study published by the Journal of Oleo Science, the anti-inflammatory properties of myrrh essential oil were examined, with the following results: "This study was designed to investigate the anti-inflammatory and antinociceptive activities of essential oil recipe (OR)…These data demonstrated that the OR inhibits inflammatory and peripheral inflammatory pain. These results may support the fact that the essential oil of traditional Hui prescription played a role in the inflammation of stroke."

This study aimed to assess the efficacy of an essential oil blend on pain and inflammation. The blend of essential oils combined white pepper, long pepper, cinnamon, saffron, and myrrh. The oral administration of the essential oil blend resulted in a reduction of ear vasodilatation in the mice tested, which results in the widening of blood vessels and a reduction in blood pressure. The oil blend also reduced the writhing that was induced by an acetic acid injection. The antinociceptive properties (receptivity to pain) and anti-inflammatory properties demonstrated by the oils reveal a potential for applying this oil blend to support pain and inflammation.

Reference
http://www.ncbi.nlm.nih.gov/pubmed/25263165]

https://www.jstage.jst.go.jp/article/jos/63/12/63_ess1406
1/_pdf

Study 3 – Sun Protection

In this study available on PubMed, the effects of myrrh essential oil in relation to skin physiology were examined, with the following results: "Squalene is a component of sebum. Both are directly exposed to the external environment and play a key role in skin physiology. They are particularly prone to photo oxidation during sun exposure. We studied the impact of two types of antioxidant on sebum squalene peroxidation by UV irradiation. The first type is free radical scavenger (Butyl hydroxyl toluene and an olive extract rich in hydroxytyrosol). The second type is the essential oil of Commipora myrrha, a singlet oxygen quencher…Our results clearly show that essential oil of Commiphora myrrha provides the best protection against squalene peroxidation. These results demonstrate that squalene peroxidation during solar exposure is mainly because of singlet oxygen and not due to free radical attack. This suggests that sun care cosmetics should make use not only of free radical scavengers but also of singlet oxygen quenchers."

The study examined the antioxidant effects of myrrh essential oil in relation to sun exposure, UV irradiation, and skin physiology. Myrrh essential oil provided significant protection against singlet oxygen, which causes damaging effects on a number of organic materials through sunlight. In this way, myrrh is an anti-agent working against the peroxidation of squalene, which is a natural moisturizer and one of the most common lipids created by human skin cells. Peroxidation is when free radicals take electrons from cell membranes, which results in the oxidative degradation of lipids and significant cell damage. This causes a chain reaction, because whenever a normal cell is in contact with a radical, another radical is produced, which means the radicals begin to multiply at an exponential rate, the end result being carcinogenic or mutagenic. The results of the study indicate that myrrh demonstrates potential in the arena of skin care and cosmetics when it comes to sun protection.

Reference
http://www.ncbi.nlm.nih.gov/pubmed/18489308]

Study 4 – Antimicrobial & Anti-infective Activity

In this study published by Letters in Applied Microbiology, the antimicrobial and anti-infective activity of myrrh essential oil was examined, with the following results: "The in vitro antimicrobial activity of three essential oil samples of frankincense (Boswellia rivae, Boswellia neglecta and Boswellia papyrifera) and two essential oil samples of myrrh and sweet myrrh (Commiphora guidotti and Commiphora myrrha), collected from different regions of Ethiopia, was investigated independently and in combination to determine their anti-infective properties…Frankincense and myrrh essential oils have been used in combination since 1500 BC; however, no antimicrobial investigations have been undertaken to confirm their effect in combination. This study validates the enhanced efficacy when used in combination against a selection of pathogens."

The objective of this study was to identify the anti-infectious and antimicrobial activity of frankincense and myrrh essential oils. Among the yeast and bacteria tested were Cryptococcus neoformans, Pseudomonas aeruginosa, and Bacillus cereus.

Cryptococcus neoformans is a yeast that, when pathogenic, is termed cryptococcosis. Infections resulting from C. neoformans often occur in the lungs, but encephalitis and fungal meningitis are also caused by C.

neoformans, which makes this yeast particularly fatal to those with damaged immune systems.

Pseudomonas aeruginosa is also a common bacteria found in water, soil, skin flora, and in man-made environments. The bacterium thrives on moist surfaces, and so can threaten the hospital environment by finding its home on medical equipment, like catheters, resulting in cross-infection. It is, for instance, the bacterium which causes hot-tub rash. This bacterium also attacks immunocompromised patients, infecting the urinary tract, airway, wounds, burns, and resulting in blood infections.

Bacillus cereus is an endemic, Gram-positive bacterium that dwells in the soil, and certain strains can cause foodborne illness. It's sometimes called "fried rice syndrome," due to the fact that this bacteria is commonly contracted from fried rice that's been left out for hours on end (like at a buffet).

Myrrh essential oil was most active against C. neoformans and P. aeruginosa, and also demonstrated synergistic effects with frankincense against B. cereus. These results indicate the efficacy of applying myrrh essential oil to the infectious bacterial and fungi strains tested.

Reference
http://www.ncbi.nlm.nih.gov/pubmed/22288378]

Study 5 – Antibacterial Properties

In this study published in Applied Microbiology and Biotechnology, the antibacterial effects of myrrh essential oil were examined, with the following results: "The long-term usage of antibiotics has resulted in the evolution of multidrug-resistant bacteria. Unlike antibiotics, anti-virulence approaches target bacterial virulence without affecting cell viability, which may be less prone to develop drug resistance. Staphylococcus aureus is a major human pathogen that produces diverse virulence factors, such as α-toxin, which is hemolytic. Also, biofilm formation of S. aureus is one of the mechanisms of its drug resistance. In this study, anti-biofilm screening of 83 essential oils showed that black pepper, cananga, and myrrh oils and their common constituent cis-nerolidol at 0.01 % markedly inhibited S. aureus biofilm formation…This finding implies other beneficial effects of essential oils and suggests that black pepper, cananga, and myrrh oils have potential use as anti-virulence strategies against persistent S. aureus infections."

The objective of this study was to evaluate the antibacterial effects of dozens of essential oils – including myrrh – on S. aureus. S. aureus is Gram-positive bacterium. Methicillin-resistant Staphylococcus aureus (MRSA) is any strain of S. aureus which has naturally developed a resistance to antibiotics, including penicillin. This hospital-acquired infection is now limitedly endemic. Being resistant to standard medications, this strain – although not more virulent than other S. aureus strains – may result in infections that are tough to treat. Hospitals, nursing homes, and prisons largely house MRSA, and patients with weak immune systems and open wounds are most at risk.

The study showed that myrrh essential oil was one of the three most active oils to inhibit S. aureus. These results further demonstrate myrrh's strong antibacterial activity and, moreover, indicate that the essential oil could potentially be used in hospitals to combat drug-resistant strains of this bacteria.

Reference
http://www.ncbi.nlm.nih.gov/pubmed/25027570]

Study 6 – Antibacterial Properties

In this study available on PubMed, the antibacterial effects of myrrh essential oil were examined, with the following results: "The chemical composition of essential oils of cabreuva (Myrocarpus fastigiatus Allemao, Fabaceae) from Brazil, cedarwood (Juniperus ashei, Cupressaceae) from Texas, Juniper berries (Juniperus communis L., Cupressaceae) and myrrh (Commiphora myrrha (Nees) Engl., Burseraceae) were analyzed using GC/FID and GC/MS…The volatile oils exhibited considerable inhibitory effects against all tested organisms, except Pseudomonas, using both test methods. Higher activity was observed against Gram-positive strains in comparison with Gram-negative bacteria."

This study, again, tested myrrh essential oil against eleven different Gram-positive and Gram-negative bacterial strains of bacteria. The strains are unlisted in the abstract; however, it is noted that food poisoning and spoilage bacteria, as well as animal and plant pathogens, were tested. The results indicate that all oils demonstrated inhibitory effects against the bacteria tested, apart from Pseudomonas. This confirms the antibacterial potential of myrrh essential oil.

Reference
http://www.ncbi.nlm.nih.gov/pubmed/20922991]

Chapter 4:
The Ins & Outs of Essential Oils

Where do essential oils come from?

Plants and plant species naturally produce essential oils for various reasons, one being to draw pollinator insects to them, another being to repel invading organisms (bacteria, animals). A number of chemical compounds compose each plant's essential oil, and the combination of these compounds is specific to each oil, which then instills in the oil its own unique properties. Essential oils can be harnessed from all sorts of plant components, including flowers, leaves, bark, fruit, roots, and resin. For instance, cinnamon oil is harnessed from bark, lemon oil from the peel, and lavender oil from lavender flowers. Certain plants can produce a few chemical variants of the same essential oil, which are acquired from different parts of the plant. Some of these parts produce a large amount of oil, while others produce just a smidgen. The oil's quality and potency depends upon a number of factors, including the subspecies of the plant, its soil conditions, the time of year and even the time of day you harvest it.

How are essential oils extracted?

Essential oils can be extracted from plants through various methods, including pressing, distillation, solvent and maceration. Let's take a brief look at each:

Pressing Method

Commonly used with citrus fruit, the pressing method extracts the oil through a technique which involves pushing the fruit peels through a press. Oily fruits and plants are best suited for this technique. Orange oil, for example, is extracted from orange skins through the pressing method.

Distillation Method

This technique harkens back to the days of old-timey moonshiners, as the same sort of method used to create strong liquor can be used to extract essential oils. Using a still, boiled water and plant materials will create steam which is then cooled by coils and condensed into a combination of water and oil. This combination doesn't mix, so the oil can then be extracted from it.

Solvent Method

Through a multi-step process, certain plant and flower oils can be extracted using alcohol and other solvents, which extort the essential oil from the plant materials.

Maceration Method

When a "carrier" or fixed oil or lard is mixed with the plant material and set out in the sun, over a period of time, the carrier oil is infused with the plant's essence. Heat sources, other than the sun, are often used to speed the process. Throughout the process, more plant material is added to produce a more potent oil.

How do you use essential oils?

Although some studies about the effectiveness of essential oils are conducted by small companies or even individuals, a number of them are conducted by the food and cosmetic industries. In general, the pharmaceutical industry shows next to no interest in herbal medicine, primarily because there are few options to patent such products. Being as such, the product's lack of profitability results in a lack of research funding. Regardless, the historical uses of essential oils tell us what we need to know: these oils have been effectively administered for centuries. The therapeutic qualifications of essential oils can be plotted in the survival of the human race across cultures and generations.

Another reason that studies on essential oils have not resulted in much conclusive evidence as to their overall effectiveness is because definitive results are sometimes difficult to prove, as the quality of each batch of oil can vary for a number of reasons. One is that essential oils are impossible to standardize. As mentioned above, even the slightest variance in soil conditions and the time of harvesting – as well as innumerable other factors – will produce a different product quality and potency. In addition, essential oils are often obtained from various species of the same plant; Eucalyptus radiata and Eucalyptus globulus can both be used in the making of therapeutic-grade eucalyptus oil and, as a result, they may have slightly different properties and degrees of strength or effectiveness.

Just as there are a number of methods by which to extract essential oils, there are a number of methods to administer them therapeutically. The variety of chemical compounds in each essential oil means that their benefits and applications also vary across the board. Below are a few of these methods.

Topical Administration

Direct application of many essential oils works like a sponge, as skin sops up chemicals and other things (like sunlight, for instance). Topical application is best when you want to clear up an ailment on the skin's surface or in the underlying muscle tissue. When applying topically, you may either massage the oil into the skin or simply dab on the skin for therapeutic results. You might combine the essential oil with a carrier oil for topical use in order to dilute its potency. This is safer, as the oil is so concentrated. You may support your body's defenses against rash or muscle pain in this manner, but you should always test your patient for allergies before applying. Adverse effects are produced by natural chemicals as much as synthetic ones; poison ivy, for example.

To test for allergens, place a drop or two on your patient's inner forearm. If a rash develops within 12 to 24 hours, then the patient is allergic. In addition, phototoxicity – sun exposure resulting in an exacerbated burn – may be an issue when citrus oils are applied topically. So one must proceed with caution when applying essential oils using this method.

Inhalation Therapy

Commonly known as "aromatherapy", this essential oil application is effective for inner ailments, like sore throat or cold. In a steaming bowl of distilled or sterilized water, add a few drops of essential oil and, with a towel over your head, bend over the bowl and inhale. The towel captures the vapors, making the technique even more effective. Essential oils can also be placed in a diffuser or potpourri throughout a room to produce somewhat diluted therapeutic effects.

Ingestion

When using this method, proceed with caution. Direct ingestion of essential oils must be monitored and applied in small doses that are diluted in a tablespoon or more of any carrier oil – olive oil, for example. If you are unsure of dosage amounts, make a tea with the relevant herb instead. Although the effects of this diluted use may be weaker, this application is a better alternative than an overdose of essential oils.

What are the general benefits of using essential oils?

Replacement for Prescription Drugs

One practical benefit for using essential oils is, of course, their substitutive nature; they can replace Rx drugs, which is the ultimate reason to educate yourself on their administration and to begin stockpiling your essential oil supply. One of the potential threats of economic or social collapse is the lack of resources, and primarily the inability to procure prescription drugs. Being as such, finding suitable supplements should be a priority when preparing for the worst.

Their portability is also a major bonus when it comes to survival prepping. The fact that these ultra-concentrated oils take up little-to-no space makes toting them to your shelter all the simpler should the need arise. And, because essential oils are highly concentrated, the application used in most methods of administration requires only a drop or two of oil, which means that tiny bottle will be long-lasting.

Cost Effective Supplement

Though money may be the last thing on your mind when it comes to prepping for a survival situation (money may even be obsolete in the event of social collapse), it is worth noting that the expense of essential oils pales in comparison to prescription drugs. Essential oils are a cost effective supplement to prescription medicine.

No Expiration Date

Another benefit of essential oils is that they do not expire, neither do they have "proper storage" requirements. A number of medicines and medicinal products must be replaced every couple years, so this sets essential oils ahead of the pack when it comes to shelf life.

Versatility

Essential oils also offer great versatility. Apart from providing therapeutic benefits, essential oils can be repurposed for household and hygienic applications. For instance, if you're looking for something that might serve your dental hygiene needs in a time of crisis, the protective oil blend is your go-to essential oil. If you want to maintain your skin's tone and condition, frankincense and lavender will do the trick; the latter also serves as sunscreen, so you can inhibit sun damage as well.

When it comes to the house or shelter, you can use essential oils to deodorize, which will come in handy in a disaster scenario where things might start to smell fishy due to lack of proper utilities and care. For example, after the 2011 tsunami and the subsequent nuclear reactor meltdown in Japan, a nurse named Risa Nakahira used essential oils to deodorize and sanitize putrid public bathrooms in overpopulated evacuation facilities. As relief workers searched for survivors, often wading through debris and decay, Nakahira also deodorized their boots and masks using essential oils. The possibilities of these natural oils are endless.

They are also versatile when it comes to the range of patients they're capable of supporting. The wellness of everyone from your great grandfather to your infant baby can be fortified with the aid of essential oils in the appropriate dosage. They even come in handy when supporting the wellness of livestock or pets. From teething infants to dementia in the elderly, from teenagers with acne to dogs with urinary tract infections, essential oils can serve any patient with nearly any ailment.

Conclusion

Now that you know all about what myrrh essential oil can do for you – where it originates, how it's extracted, its benefits and properties, and the different methods of administration – you can use it confidently to support the body's defenses against health issues and start to assemble a kit of essential oils for survival. Essential oils can be purchased online or at your local holistic treatment store.

The various benefits of essential oils and their properties are countless. To build your own kit, first focus on acquiring the essential oils which may bear more relevance to your health issues or the potential health threats within your environment. When it comes to skin health, for instance, myrrh essential oil will be one of your more crucial oils, due to its antibacterial, anti-inflammatory, antifungal, and astringent properties.

Used as a supplement or as your go-to for immune system support, blood circulation, or gum and hair health, the application of myrrh essential oil in medicine has survived for centuries and will survive centuries more. When it comes down to it, you don't need to rely on pharmaceuticals; essential oils, herbs, and plenty of other natural ingredients can be used to help support any number of health issues, whether ailment or injury.

Essential oils are essential to your survival in the case of viral outbreak, social collapse or natural disaster because, when the SHTF, your access to pharmaceuticals will likely either be limited or eliminated altogether. Alternatives to our modern-day standard will equate survival when no other option exists. And when it comes to a life-or-death situation, you can't let your health decline, no matter the state of the world.

DISCLAIMER AND/OR LEGAL NOTICES: Every effort has been made to accurately represent this book and it's potential. Results vary with every individual, and your results may or may not be different from those depicted. No promises, guarantees or warranties, whether stated or implied, have been made that you will produce any specific result from this book. Your efforts are individual and unique, and may vary from those shown. Your success depends on your efforts, background and motivation.

The material in this publication is provided for educational and informational purposes only and is not intended as medical advice. The information contained in this book should not be used to diagnose or treat any illness, metabolic disorder, disease or health problem. Always consult your physician or healthcare provider before beginning any nutrition or exercise program. Use of the programs, advice, and information contained in this book is at the sole choice and risk of the reader.